PATELLOFEMORAL KNEE SYNDROME

A complete guide to defeat patellofemoral knee syndrome

TABLE OF CONTENTS

INTRODUCTION

The patellofemoral joint, a part of the knee joint complex has been often defined as one of the most investigated small joints in the body, developing pain and inability far out of proportion to its size.

Patellofemoral problems are highly widespread in sports athletes and can result in chronic pain, lack of stability, weakness, and irregular or weak athletic performance. These problems could be hard to identify. Treatment choices may vary depending on various factors, such as the sport and the time throughout the sports season when the signs and symptoms appear. Treatment may also differ according to the age of the patient and their level of competition.

Patellofemoral Knee syndrome offers an in depth review of the physical examination, radiographic analysis, differential medical determinations, and treatment choices of typical patellofemoral diseases, such as patellar chondrosis, pain and unbalances. The contributors are nationwide, known professionals in the patella femoral joint that deal with athletes of every age group. This book is an extensive manual for the distinctive and sport specific problems of athletes of every age and expertise regarding the patellofemoral joint.

The high occurrence of patellofemoral pain makes this a must read discourse for any generalist and practitioner. It's also a useful source of information for physiotherapists.

Copyright 2014 by RustburgStuff

All rights reserved.

CHAPTER 1

COMMON KNEE INJURIES

In this chapter you will learn about;

- ➢ Patellofemoral knee syndrome
- ➢ ACL Tear
- ➢ Meniscus Tear
- ➢ Osteoarthritis

For many of us, knee injuries often occur out of the blue, or they find their way up certainly as time passes. But the truth is there are actually things all sports athletes and fitness enthusiasts can do to prevent the possibility of knee injuries.

The different forms of injuries to the knee are characterized by the affected anatomy of the knee and the process during which it is damaged.

PATELLOFEMORAL PAIN SYNDROME

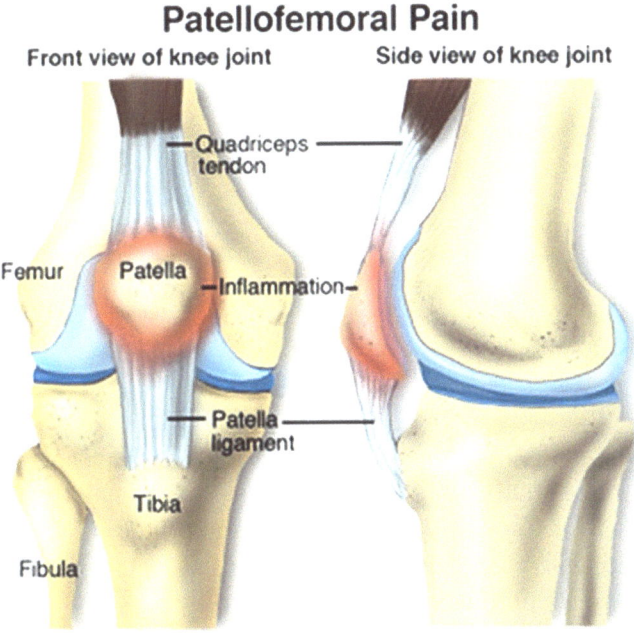

Patellofemoral pain syndrome is characterized by pain experienced behind the kneecap. Walking up and down the stairs, squatting, or sitting still for prolonged durations can worsen the pain. The normal cause is abnormal movement of the kneecap as the knee is bent and straightened out. This may result in damage of the cartilage on the back of the kneecap. Fluctuations in muscle strength, tight muscles, and structural problems of the lower rimb can add to the problem. The pain normally occurs slowly but surely eventually.

ANTERIOR CRUCIATE LIGAMENT (ACL TEAR)

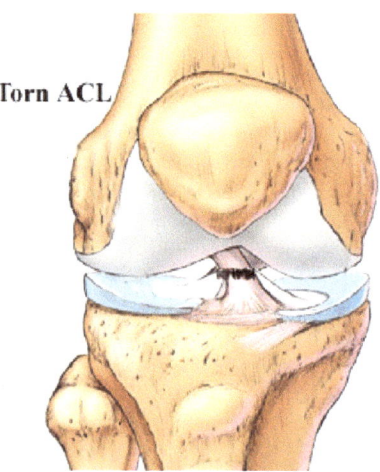

Torn ACL

Normally, this is a non contact injury and often consists of flexion, valgus, and external rotation. Typically a "pop" is felt; the sufferer is unable to continue specific activities, and needs to be helped to the sideline. It is actually a critical injury with large effusion that gets worse in a single day.

The sufferer walks for about a week with bent knee limp and seems fairly normal by three weeks. Meniscal injuries also appear with ACL tears about 60-70 % of the time. Other ligament injuries arise 10-15 % of the time.

DEGENERATIVE MENISCUS TEAR

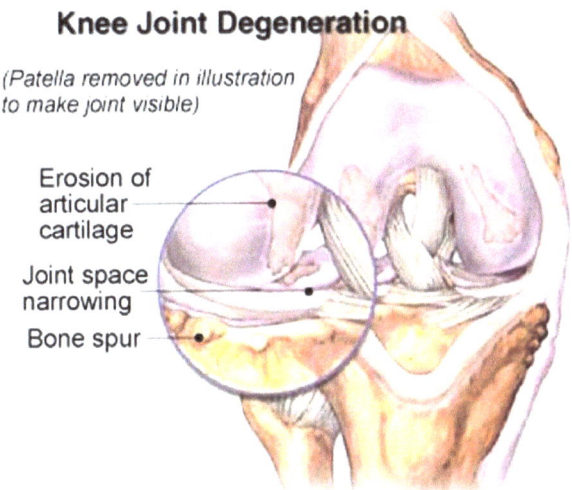

Knee Joint Degeneration

(Patella removed in illustration to make joint visible)

Erosion of articular cartilage

Joint space narrowing

Bone spur

Degenerative meniscus tears usually appear in men over 40 years old or women over 50 years old. Pain is normally at the center medial part of the joint line or lateral joint line, often brought on by a twisting injury, but can take place without injury. It may also have locking of the knee. Traumatic meniscal tears rise in the young people taking part in high-risk exercises with joint line pain on the side of the tear, and also swelling and locking.

OSTEOARTHRITIS

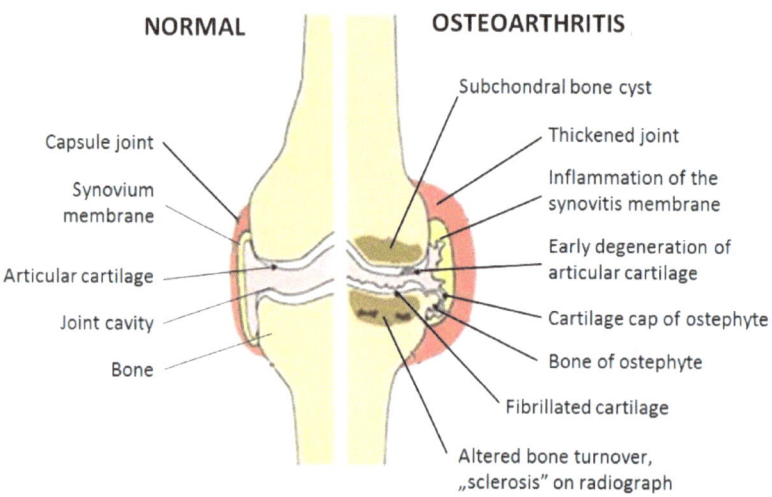

This injury normally takes place in people over 60 years old, until there's a background of meniscal tear treated with meniscectomy and then can take place in people in their twenties or fifties. There could be mild pain with a diverse amount of effusion. If it is in an area of focal pain, then consider other medical diagnosis, for example meniscal tear, either by itself or in combination. Other factors are a threatening onset with ultimate limited motion, and pain worse with extended standing and walking and higher pain with stairs, particularly if patellofemoral element is engaged.

CHAPTER 2

PATELLOFEMORAL PAIN SYNDROME

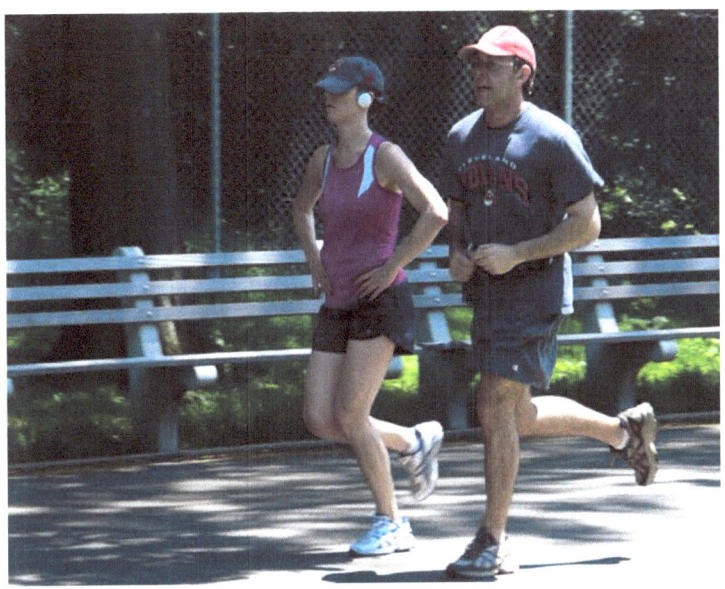

In this chapter you will learn about;

- ➢ Patella

- ➢ Functions of Patella

- ➢ Femur

- ➢ Symptoms of PFPS

Patellofemoral pain syndrome is the term related to pain originated from patella when the patella contacts with the femur. This pain is common in athletes and manual labor. Patellofemoral pain syndrome accounts for several sports related knee injuries. There are many factors that affect this pain syndrome such as soft tissue tightness, muscle weakness and excessive exercise or running that's why the Patellofemoral pain syndrome is multi-factorial in origin.

Clinical treatment of the Patellofemoral pain syndrome is challenging due to multiple factors affecting Patellofemoral joint. The most effective treatment of anterior is the physical rehab programs, because this physical rehabilitation program is non operative option.

Patellofemoral pain syndrome arises when a person suffering from knee disorder sits on knees for a long time, performs the squat exercise, jumps, and goes down the stairs or excessive cycling in an inappropriate manner.

PATELLA

The Patella is a circular and a little triangular thicker bone and is the largest sesamoid bone in the human body and lies within the quadriceps tendons. It is also known as kneecap or kneepan and covers or protects the anterior articular surface of the knee. The front of the patella is covered with bursa (*a small fluid-filled sac located between movable parts of the body, especially at joints and there are 14 different bursae with respect to three different sides of the knee: frontal side, lateral side and medial side*) and the back of the patella is covered with soft or smooth bone called cartilage that helps in straightening your leg by assisting the patella to slide over the femur (a lower part of the thigh bone).

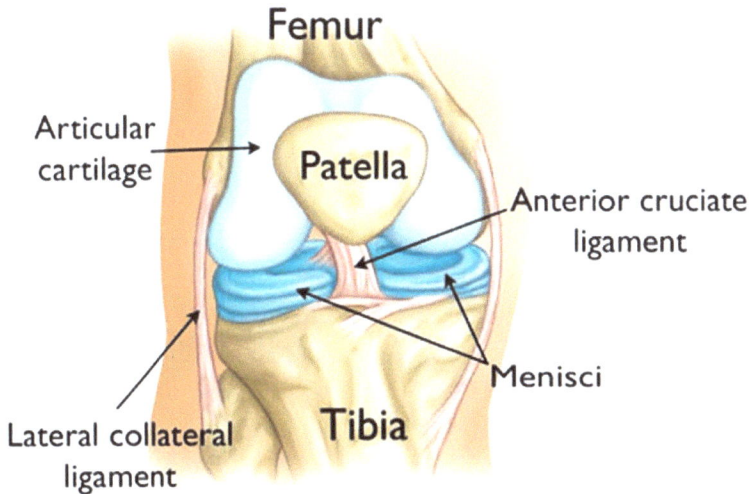

Patella has two surfaces anterior and posterior. Anterior surface has three parts and the posterior surface has two (2) parts. The Patella is responsible for proper functioning of our knee as it is connected or attached to the tendons of the quadriceps muscle (femoris) that contract for extending and straighten our knee.

PATELLOFEMORAL KNEE SYNDROME

Our patella increases the power to act effectively and in response our tendons attached to it exerts force on the femur in order to perform the desired function.

The disorder in patella structure may result in disturbance in knee extension or pain while doing healthy activities or normal routine activities as well. The chances of disorders such as patellar dislocation in patella are more in athlete women than men. In patella dislocation our patella slides out of its original position often in a lateral direction and can cause swelling or severe pain.

FUNCTIONS OF PATELLA

Patella's primary function is knee extension or flexion efficiency and to protect or cover the tibiofemoral joint. Patella along with other tendons and muscles make knee correct movement possible.

FEMUR

Femur is the thigh bone and being a bone it provides support to our body during different standing positions and also helps in different movements of our legs such as walking, jumping and running. It is the longest and strongest bone of our body. The distal (situated farthest from the point of attachment or origin, as of a limb or bone) part of the femur form knee joint by joining with the tibia (a lower leg bone) and patella or kneecap.

SYMPTOMS OF PFPS

There are many symptoms of Patellofemoral pain syndrome or pain related to our knees such as pain around the knee or at the front of the kneecap. In most of the cases, knee pain is often felt approximately at the front of the knee.

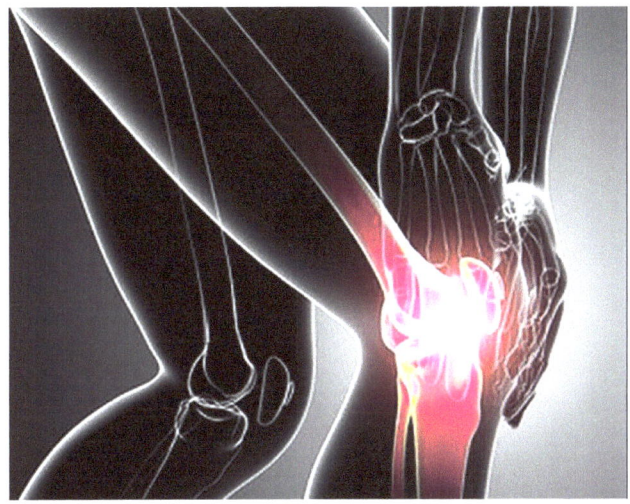

Here are some symptoms prescribed by the majority of the physicians and arthropathy specialists;

• Feeling pain at the front of the knee sometimes in the form of severe pain. This pain can be felt when a load is put on the knee while kneeling, cycling excessively or running

• Patellofemoral pain can be felt in different intervals, because this pain comes and goes

• Patellofemoral pain can be felt vaguely while practicing knee exercises with high intensity, because in some knee exercises the heavy load is mainly put on the knee extensor mechanism

• Feeling pain while going down the stairs or during squat exercises while lifting heavy weight

• The prolonged sitting with bent knees can also results Patellofemoral pain syndrome

• Joint noises called crepitus such as grinding feeling during the movement of knee joint

• Feeling pain in knee along with swelling

These symptoms are not enough to diagnose Patellofemoral pain syndrome alone, because there are many other ways of determining this pain such as X-ray and scans. Although X-rays and scans are not helpful in diagnosing the Patellofemoral pain syndrome, but these methods are used to look for other knee conditions such as fractures and broken tendons.

CHAPTER 3

CAUSES OF PATELLOFEMORAL PAIN SYNDROME

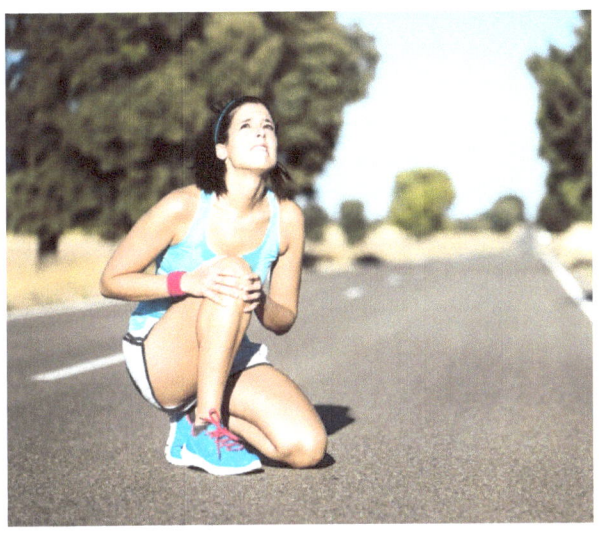

Our body is designed to perform several physiological and mental activities. These activities regulate our body systems and generate energy for the proper functioning of voluntary and involuntary organs as well. Our body contains several joints along with tissues related to these joints. These tissues and joints work together in order to perform different movements such as walking, sitting, kneeling, running, swimming, climbing and lifting heavy objects. Moving body parts (organs) in a moderate manner and gradually increasing intensity of physical activities, is a healthy way of keeping running your body.

These activities like exercising if done in high intensity much more intense than our physical abilities can develop many health issues especially related to muscles and joints. Some of these health problems are not easy to diagnose and treat like complex joint pain syndromes such as Patellofemoral pain syndrome (PFPS) or knee pain syndrome.

Knee pain can be felt due to different disorders or diseases that lead or provoke anterior knee pain such as osteoarthritis, iliotibial band friction syndrome, medial overload syndrome, Hoffa's fad syndrome, hip joint disorder and patellar tendinitis etc.

These all factors are not Patellofemoral pain syndrome, but can cause knee pain. There are multiple factors of Patellofemoral pain syndrome that cause this pain. Due to the combination of different factors Patellofemoral pain syndrome has several causes. Some of the most common causes are described below in order to accurately understand knee pain syndrome;

- The most common cause of knee pain syndrome that has been seen in athletes, is over use of knee or practicing too hard or too much such as running and squatting that cause rubbing of the patella over femur and also cause physiological mal-alignment of the lower extremities especially in the knee joint

- Prolonged sitting under unfavorable conditions like prolonged sitting with knees bent

- Weak hip and thigh muscles

- Knee alignment: it has been seen that knee alignment can cause the patella rubbing over the femur instead of gliding. This alignment is generally caused by the imbalance in muscle strength around the knee. Dysfunction of patella gliding over the femur is caused by imbalance in quadriceps muscles

- Running on a hard rough track for a long time can cause Patellofemoral pain syndrome

- Putting excessive strain on knees through prolonged wearing shoes with hard soles and walking while lifting heavy weight for long period

- Weak muscles that support patella movement around the knee also cause knee syndrome

- Too tight or too loose ligaments and tendons often cause knee syndrome or Patellofemoral pain syndrome

- Weakness in the medial quadriceps causes

- Over weight and obesity often lead to joint healthy issues and is also a cause of Patellofemoral knee/pain syndrome. Our excessive weight put extra strain on our knees especial when we are having some physical activities while on knees

- Injury during sports related to knee excessive workouts can cause knee syndrome

- A pushed kneecap outer side of the knee joint due to a forceful blow causes knee syndrome

- Flat feet: a foot afflicted with a fallen arch; abnormally flattened and spread out. Flatfoot is associated with the lower part of the legs being angled outward and leads mal-alignment of patella or knee joint

- Tight iliotibial band exerts/stresses more than adequate lateral force on the patella and thus it disturbs the Patellofemoral mechanism. Sometimes tight iliotibial band also rotate the tibia externally and leads to (PFPS)

- Hip dysfunction , loose ligaments, poorly aligned bones and overload knee joint are some common causes that lead to knee pain syndrome

CHAPTER 4

DIAGNOSIS AND TREATMENTS

In this chapter you will learn about;

- ➢ Diagnosis of knee syndrome
- ➢ Treatment of Patellofemoral Pain syndrome
- ➢ Surgical treatments (operative)
- ➢ Non operative treatments
- ➢ Physiotherapy
- ➢ Patellar taping
- ➢ Initial treatment
- ➢ Flexibility or stretching workouts
- ➢ Preventions and precautionary measures

DIAGNOSIS OF KNEE SYNDROME

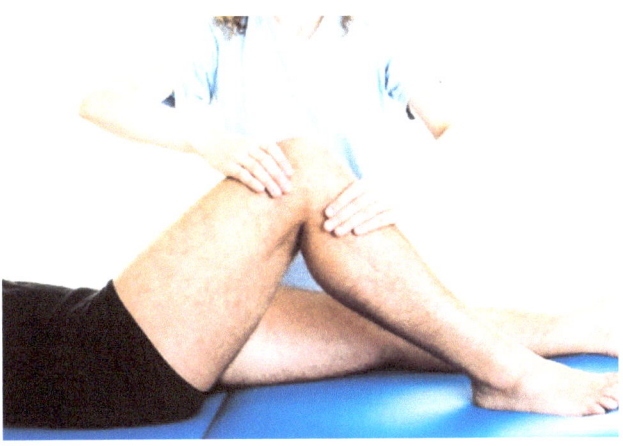

Due to the multiple factors, Patellofemoral pain syndrome or knee syndrome cannot be diagnosed in simple ways. The diagnosis of knee syndrome can be made through the symptoms and a thorough examination of the retinacular structure around the knee (patella). A radiograph of patella can be helpful in diagnosing knee syndrome.

TREATMENT OF PATELLOFEMORAL PAIN SYNDROME

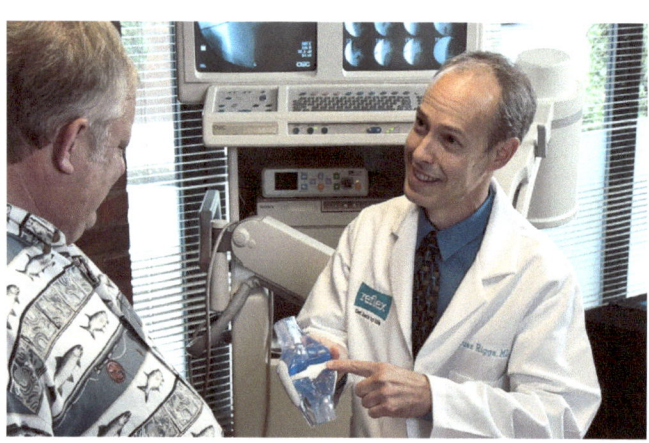

Patellofemoral pain syndrome is a complex pain caused by several factors described in earlier chapters. Knee is very important part of our body that allows us to perform several activities such as walking, running, sitting and other knee related activities. Therefore, we need to treat our knee carefully in order to prevent knee syndrome.

If someone has suffered from knee pain, then he or she needs to avoid all activities that put great strain on knees such as intense workouts while on knees, squatting, cycling walking, and running going down or up long distance stairs. Prolonged sitting also makes Patellofemoral pain syndrome worse than before, so we need to avoid all these activities that make this pain worse. I am not asking you to leave your fitness, just avoid, or reduce the activities that can make your pain worse.

Patellofemoral pain syndrome can be treated by surgical (operative) and non surgical (non operative) treatments.

SURGICAL TREATMENTS (OPERATIVE)

In surgical treatment, surgery is performed to realign or restore patella tracking to normal conditions. Surgery is not needed for all health conditions of Patellofemoral pain syndrome; it is needed only in severe healthy conditions of knee. Surgery is also needed to treat tight ligament.

Surgery is recommended to those who do not care about their knee pain in the beginning when it hurts a little bit and ignores other healthy ways to treat their knee pain syndrome.

NON OPERATIVE TREATMENTS

There are many ways to treat patella femoral pain syndrome due to its multiple factors causing this knee pain syndrome. Non operative or non surgical treatments are considered effective in most of patients of Patellofemoral pain syndrome such as (physiotherapy) balanced strengthening, hip external rotator strengthening, quadriceps muscle stretching exercises, proprioceptive (relating to proprioception), foot orthoses, patellar taping and effective bracing. These treatments are considered best way to avoid surgery and medications (taking painkillers on regular basis).

PHYSIOTHERAPY

Exercise, massage and other modalities to treat injured muscles and joints related to these muscles or vice versa are called physiotherapy. Physiotherapy for treating Patellofemoral pain syndrome strengthens muscles around the knee (patella). Physiotherapy is also used to treat muscle imbalance and alignment that cause knee pain syndrome. In physiotherapy specific physical activities (specially designed exercises or conditioning program) are asked to practice in order to strengthen the inner muscles that are weak or cause knee pain.

PATELLAR TAPING

The inexpensive self management strategy used to treat knee pain syndrome. Patellar taping corrects displacement of patella (due to multiple factors) by creating mechanical realignment. Taping is also effective in morning stiffness, difficulty in doing routine works/tasks, instability of joints and knee pain syndrome. Patella taping reduces pain immediately; it increases knee flexion while walking with variable speed and going up and down the stairs. It has been seen that medial patellar taping give a radiographic positional change of the patella especially in the people suffered from Patellofemoral pain syndrome.

REST THE KNEE (INITIAL TREATMENT)

Our natural healing system works all the time especially when we are sleeping after doing some healthy physical activities. The people suffering from severe knee pain due to Patellofemoral pain syndrome must take rest for a few days in order to repair their knee through natural healing system. Resting doesn't mean that you are asked to leave all healthy activities good for your knee and not to consult a doctor. Do all what you can do for the betterment of your knee, but avoid all those unhealthy activities that can make your pain worse.

FLEXIBILITY OR STRETCHING WORKOUTS

Patellofemoral pain syndrome involve several factors such as muscle weakness related to knee joint and knee movements like Calf, hip, thigh, tight hamstrings and iliotibial band are responsible for different knee movements and weakness or dysfunction of these muscles can cause Patellofemoral pain syndrome.

Flexibility exercises like stretching of these muscles is too much important and useful in Patellofemoral pain syndrome. Stretching your muscles related to your knee joints prevent from surgery and also relieve from pain in quicker short time. Stretching exercises along with muscle strengthening workouts improve muscles strength and joint quality and performance.

PREVENTIONS AND PRECAUTIONARY MEASURES

"Prevention is better than cure" is a well know proverb that realizes us the importance of prevention and abstention and also makes us aware of the dangers of having surgery to cure your knee. Those who do not care properly of their knee pain syndrome by having other physiotherapeutic treatments must face severe pain in their knee and are often recommended surgery.

One more thing you must keep in your mind "self-done is well done" treat your disorders by yourself. You can do better for you than others can do for you. Try to abstain from doing all the physical activities that are hazardous to your knee or can encourage more pain and lead to worse conditions of Patellofemoral pain syndrome. Although the total prevention of Patellofemoral pain syndrome is not possible, but you can avoid all your actions possible for you in order to reduce knee pain and getting it worst than before.

Here are some tips to prevent knee pain getting worse;

- Avoid doing activities that can make your knee pain worse such as intense exercising while on knees or shifting excessive load to your knees

- Be careful while going up or down the stairs or try to avoid going up or down the stairs during the period of severe knee pain

- Always do some proper warm up before practicing fitness workouts or your professional training

- The sports persons should wear suitable and reliable footwear in order to prevent joint problems especially related to knee joints while having high intensity workouts

- Do not leave all your healthy activities that keep you fit for life and maintain your health, instead switch to other healthy activities such as running can be switched to swimming and rowing

- Do stretching exercises for your lower muscles related to knee joints along with other exercises in order to heal your knee joint pain

- Do not exercises that increase your knee pain as these exercises can make your problem worse and often lead to surgery

- Try not to take pain killers before practicing physiotherapeutic exercises for the treatment of Patellofemoral pain syndrome and other joint problems. Painkillers reduce pain and you cannot realize which exercise increases your pain and thus your injury gets worse

- Do not be excited while doing your fitness workouts or other healthy activities. In excitement, you can easily overuse your body organs and thus injure yourself

- Take great care of your injuries by icing, massaging and using other techniques that are helpful for your injuries

- Do strengthening exercises for the muscles related to sensitive joints especially in case of Patellofemoral pain syndrome

- Take some non-steroid anti-inflammatory agents prescribed by a physiotherapist or a physician in order to relieve your pain

Consult your physiotherapist, if condition of your knee is not improving with all abstentions or preventions.

CHAPTER 5

REHAB EXERCISES FOR PATELLOFEMORAL PAIN SYNDROME

In this chapter you will learn about;

- ➢ Quadriceps strengthening exercises
- ➢ Quad sets
- ➢ Ma Bu (Horse Stance) stance
- ➢ Straight Leg Raise
- ➢ Calf Raise
- ➢ Hamstring stretch
- ➢ Best stretching workouts for patellofemoral pain syndrome

Exercises increase life quality and endurance along with many other benefits. Exercising in an appropriate manner increase our muscles strength and stability. Some of the professional athletes damage their muscles and joints by overusing some body organs, joints, or muscles related to these joints. Knee pain is common in athletes or exercising people involved in running, walking and all sports related to joints especially exercises that shift load mainly to the knees and foot joints. Generally, knee pain is originated from patella when it contacts with the femur; femur is the longest and thickest bone of our skeleton that extends from the pelvis to the knee joint. This type of knee pain is known as Patellofemoral pain syndrome (PFPS).

PATELLOFEMORAL KNEE SYNDROME

Patellofemoral pain syndrome can be treated in a variety of ways by using different techniques. Most of the treatments or techniques used to treat Patellofemoral pain syndrome have described in earlier chapters. The most beneficial way to treat PFPS is physical therapy and strength workouts to improve the quality of joints and muscles related to these joints. The physiotherapeutic techniques include flexibility or stretching exercises along with some core strengthening workouts.

The strong muscles around the knee joint and responsible for knee movements can prevent knee damage during high impact workouts and can heal our knee joint in quicker short time by allowing us to perform different healthy activities (exercises).

QUADRICEPS STRENGTHENING EXERCISES

The conditioning or physical exercising program concentrating on improving thigh muscles (quadriceps and vastus medialis obliquus) has been consistently been found to be effective in reducing pain in the people suffering from Patellofemoral pain syndrome. Our quadriceps is responsible for the correct movement of our knee. Weak quadriceps results in dislocation or extra stress on the patella during running, walking and going up or down the stairs. Here are some exercises for strengthening quadriceps in case of Patellofemoral pain syndrome;

QUAD SETS

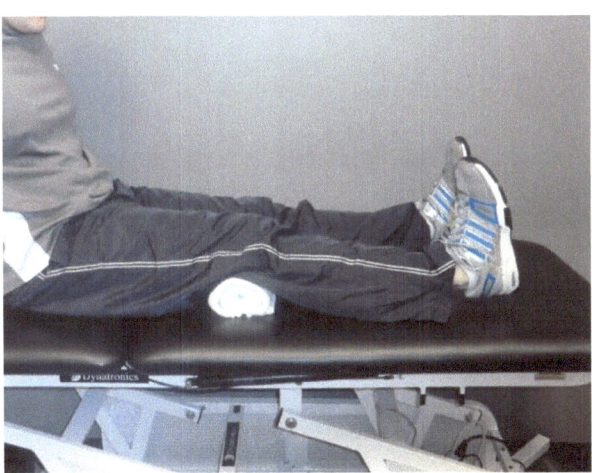

- Sit on a bench with a sufficient cushioning while resting your leg (with injured knee or knee with pain) on the bench

- Rest your both hands behind you on the bench in order to support you leg and also for balancing your body during workout

● Place a soft cushioning rolled up cloth under your affected knee joint in order to fill the gap. If the gap is not filled with a soft rolled-up cloth (a towel or something like that), then it can emphasize extra stress on your knee

● Now, tighten the front thigh muscles of affected knee and hold for 5 to 6 seconds if the condition is severe and the condition is not severe, then hold for at least 8 seconds

● After required or desired time relax your thigh muscles completely as recovery for at least 10 second or 8 seconds

● Repeat this workout for 10 to 15 minutes or according to prescription of your physiotherapist and according to the physiological condition of your knee

● Bench is not essential you can sit on the carpeted floor or can use an exercise mat while resting your hands behind your back on the floor in order to support your leg and the whole body

● Keep straight your affected leg and bent the other one and do the same workout (using a bench)

MA BU (HORSE STANCE) STANCE

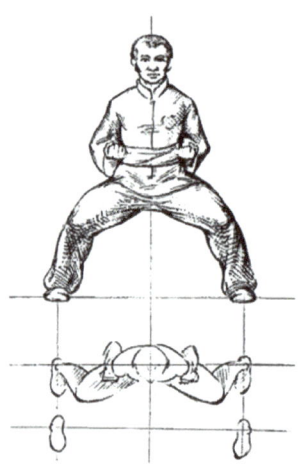

In case of, when you feel minor pain in your knee, Ma Bu position is the best exercise for strengthening your lower muscles (calf thigh muscles) and also for improving quadriceps muscles core quality. Follow these simple tips in order to correctly perform this exercise;

● Do some warm up for your legs depending on the condition of you knee and muscles related to knee joint and stretch your legs at shoulder width on a carpeted floor or on the exercise mat

● Slowly bent your knees (as torso sinks down in a straight line) while keeping your upper body straight in such a way that your knees should be bent less than 90 degree and your feet should be parallel and straight forward

● Hold this position for 5 to 6 seconds and then move to your starting point and relax for at least 10 seconds

● Repeat this workout for 3 to 4 time if your knee does not hurt during this workout

If you feel pain then avoid doing this exercise

Variations

● After a few days when you feel your knee is recovering, extend your duration of stay and after completing 3 to 4 repetitions do this exercise by slowly going down and up (do not stand completely while moving up your torso and also avoid bending your knees less than 90 degree angle)

● Adopt other rehab workouts if you feel pain during Ma Bu position or horse stance exercise

STRAIGHT LEG RAISE

Straight leg raise exercise is generally practices to strengthen thighs, hips, and abs muscles and improve the core quality of these muscles. Straight leg raise is a low impact exercise and it is generally practiced without exercising equipment as a rehab workout. The main muscle involve in this exercise are;

> Sartorius

> Pectineus

> Rectus Femoris

> Ab muscles (gets a secondary workout)

> Obliques

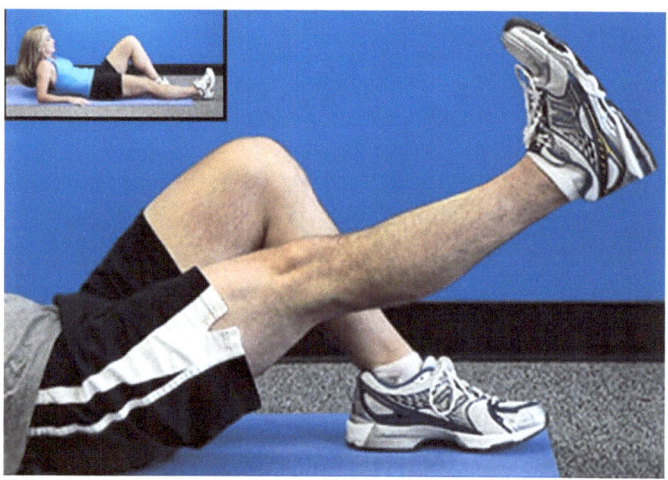

Method

Gently massage your knee with good oil with healthy effects and good penetrating quality, before you start your rehab workout and do some warm up if possible. You can move your hands and neck in circle inwards and outwards and stretch your hands. This will stimulate blood circulation throughout your body.

• Sit on a comfortable mat like exercise mat while keeping straight your both legs

• Not fold your uninvolved leg or the leg with no injured knee and keep straight your leg with injured knee or involved leg

- (1) Lean back on your elbows in order to support your body during the movement of involved leg. (2) straight leg raise can be performed in another i.e. lie on your back while keeping your leg straight with injured knee and bend the other leg with flat foot on the mat or carpeted floor with sufficient cushioning

- Pull your toes towards your face while keeping your leg straight

- Slowly raise your leg with injured knee and tighten the thigh muscles

- Hold your raised knee 6 to 7 seconds or according to the physical condition of your knee and keep it straight

- Slowly lower your leg and rest for up to 10 seconds

- Repeat this exercise 10 to 12 times or according to the prescription of your physiotherapist

CALF RAISE

Calf raise exercise strengthens our shin muscles and improves the performance of our lower body movements.

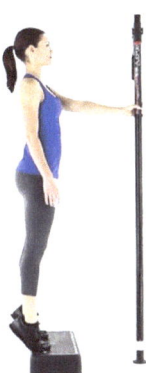

Muscles involved

The muscles involved in this exercise are;

- Tibialis anterior

- Extensor Digitorum longus

- Tibia

- Soleus muscles

- Gastrocnemius muscle

- Extensor hallucis longus

Method

• Stand near a wall while resting your hands on the wall

• Keep your face towards the wall

• Stretch your both feet equally from each other (keep distance of 1 12 inches between both your feet)

• Put equally weight on both feet and slowly raise your body with the help of your toes on the ground while lifting your heels together

• Hold you r position for 6 to 7 seconds and lower your body to the starting position slowly

• Repeat this exercise for 12 to 15 times or according to the prescription given by your physiotherapist

HAMSTRING STRETCH

Hamstring stretch improves the performance and core quality of hamstring muscles.

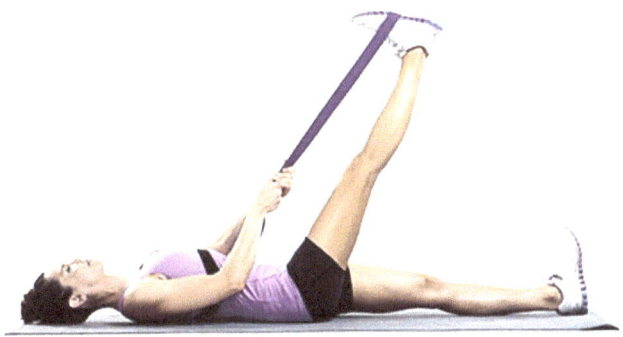

Muscles involved

Hamstring and front thigh muscles are mainly involved in this exercise.

Method

Here are some tips to perform accurately hamstring stretch;

- Lie down on your back on the exercise mat or some cushiony material in order to prevent back pain and for doing with ease and comfort

- Wrap or loop a resistance band around your feet with injured knee

- Hold the ends of resistance band firmly in both your hands

- Raise your involved leg while keeping it straight making almost 60 degree angle

- Hold this position for 15 to 20 seconds or according to the physical condition of your knee

BEST STRETCHING WORKOUTS FOR PATELLOFEMORAL PAIN SYNDROME

Stretching exercises allow your muscles related to knee joint, full range of motion and improved muscle balance. Stretching hamstring, calf, and thigh muscles reduces muscles tightness or stiffness and also reduces excessive tension on your kneecap. Stretching also helps regain full muscle length and thus it helps in relieving knee pain caused by patellofemoral pain syndrome.

Here is the method of stretching your lower body that restores full muscle length and normalizing your muscles;

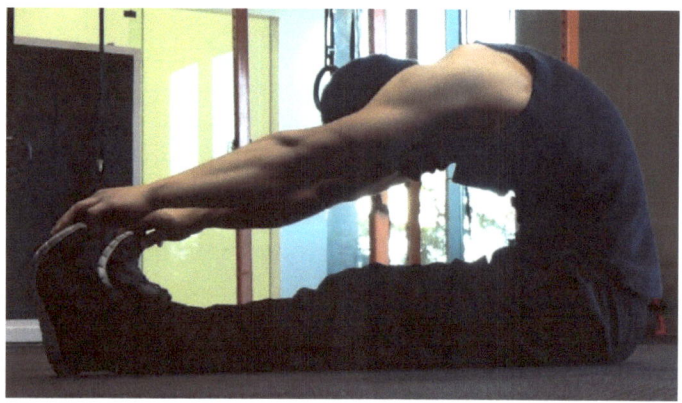

• Sit on a cushiony floor or on the exercise mat while keeping straight your both legs forward

• Make 90 degree angle between your torso and legs

• Pull your toes towards your face and try to touch your toes slowly while keeping your knees straight and moving your body towards your feet

- Try to touch your knees with your chest and keep your head straight towards your feet

- Place a rolled up towel under your knees in order to prevent knee pain

- Hold this position for 3 to 5 seconds and release your position for 3 seconds and then do it again

- Repeat this exercise for 5 to 7 minutes

CHAPTER 6

NATURAL REMEDIES TO CURE KNEE PAIN

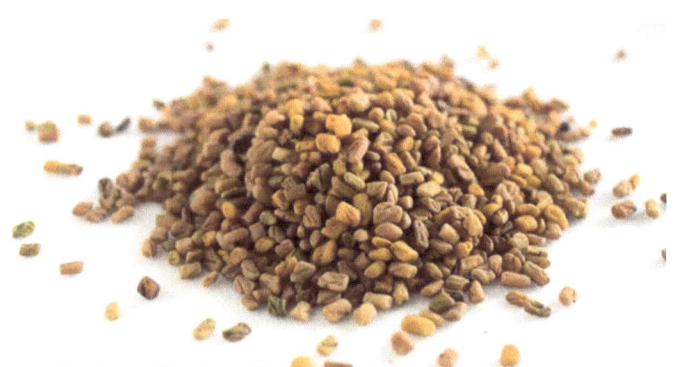

Joint Pain Relief Remedies and Natural Treatments that Work

Light to mild knee pain can be effectively treated at home. No matter whether caused by a patellofemoral knee syndrome or arthritis, there are many techniques to overcome the pain.

These natural remedies can really help reduce pain, inflammation, and stiffness:

REST: Rest the joint, and have a break from the usual activities affecting the knee joint.

ICE: Ice can relieve soreness and pain. Use ice or cold packs promptly in order to relieve or reduce inflammation. Use the ice for almost 15 minutes, 3 times a day. Lift the harmed or painful area on soft cushions while applying ice and whenever you're relaxing or lying. Keep the area at or above the level of the heart that will help reduce inflammation.

COMPRESSION: A compression bandage will help reduce inflammation and knee alignment. It shouldn't be too tight and must be taken out at nighttime.

MASSAGE: Carefully rub or massage the area to cure pain and stimulate blood circulation. Never massage the harmed area if this brings about pain.

DRINK PLENTY OF WATER: One of the lesser known advantages of consuming more water is that it softens cartilage and helps to keep it hydrated. Water can also help you keep a satisfactory blood volume so that nutrients can move through the blood and into the joints. Furthermore, it moves away wastes from the joints, which makes them less likely to ache.

GINGER EXTRACTS: Ginger is out there in various forms. It can be bought in pre-packed supplement from health food stores. Ginger root or tea is often found at the food market. This spice is used in lots of dishes. Health advantages include alleviation from stomach problems and nausea and also pain relief for several problems. A research of men and women with joint disease discovered that ginger aided to relieve pain if used along with a prescribed treatment for joint disease.

FENUGREEK: Fenugreek is really a well-known home remedy for knee pain as a result of its anti-oxidant and anti-inflammatory properties. It is especially effective for all those suffering from patellofemoral knee syndrome.

Swallow 1 teaspoon of ground fenugreek seeds and then a glass of warm water. Try this everyday in the morning till you have great results.

ONIONS: They're well-known anti-inflammatory food. They comprise phytochemicals that boost the immune system. The sulfur materials in onions hinder the enzymes that induce pain. A report confirms that fresh onions have a pain killer effect just like morphine.

Glucosamine: Glucosamine slows down cartilage damage, reduces pain, and enhances joint function. It is made out of the shells of crabs, lobsters, and shrimp.

ORTHOTICS: Orthotics, a mechanical device, is often used to support and protect arthritic joints and reduce knee pain. A brace put on an irritated joint provides pain relief by supporting the joint and reducing some of the stress brought on by body weight. Braces can also straighten joints that are being deformed. Shoes are yet another type of orthotics; soles that take up some of the shock of walking can be extremely helpful.

WILLOW BARK: A report released in 2001 discovered that some individuals with joint inflammation experienced pain alleviation using willow bark. The extract is widely used by herbal healthcare specialists to deal with high temperature, soreness, and pain.

TURMERIC: Turmeric can be a great remedy for joint pain. It has an active substance known as curcumin with anti-inflammatory and anti-oxidant properties. In a study published in 2009 in the Journal of Alternative and Complementing Medicine, experts compared the usefulness of this compound to ibuprofen and discovered that curcumin was as good as ibuprofen for pain relief in people with knee disease.

Mix 1 teaspoon of turmeric powder and a little honey in a glass of warm milk. Drink it daily for 5 days.

CAYENNE PEPPER: Cayenne pepper has a substance known as capsaicin with natural pain killing properties. In a study published in the Journal of the Medical Association of Thailand in 2010, the analysts discovered that applying gel comprising 0.0125 % capsaicin reduce light to mild pain in females affected by knee problems.

Heat 1 cup of coconut oil and mix 2 tablespoons of cayenne powder in it. Apply it around the affected area, leave it on for 25 minutes, and then wash off. Use it daily till you see an improvement.

EPSOM SALT BATHS: Epsom Salt Baths help in easy absorption of magnesium from the skin. Joint pain is usually linked to lower levels of magnesium. Furthermore, magnesium reduces swelling and helps with detoxification of cells.

Mix 2 cups Epsom salt in water bath with warm water. Bathe in it for 25 minutes, 3 times a week.

GARLIC: Being loaded with sulfur and selenium, garlic is effective for people suffering from patellofemoral knee syndrome and joint pain. Sulfur can help reduce joint pain and swelling and, in accordance with a study, selenium can have an antirheumatic effect.

Add fresh or cooked garlic in your daily diet. You can easily eat 2 or 3 garlic cloves every day. In case you're frustrated by the smell of garlic, think about garlic supplements.

Last but not least, quit smoking because smoking slows down the healing process.

CHAPTER 7

HOW TO KINESIO TAPE A PATELLA KNEE

In this chapter you will learn about;

➢ What you will need for taping

➢ Benefits of Patella Taping

➢ How to tape

➢ Removing the Tape

I suggest seeking expert advice prior to trying any self treatment. For this taping to be effective it is essential to fully grasp how the patella should be adjusted. It is often turned, tilted, and glided laterally.

FOR TAPING YOU'LL NEED

1. Kinesio tape

2. Sharp scissors

3. Things to do before Before Taping the Patella

4. How to Tape

BENEFITS OF PATELLA TAPING

When used properly, patella taping techniques can:

➢ Reduce pain during any sports activity

➢ Correct patella positioning (*Enable an earlier come back to sports activity or any other activities*)

➢ Minimize the possibility of injury aggravation

➢ Avoid knee injuries, like a dislocated patella, during sports

➢ Strengthen activation of the VMO muscle

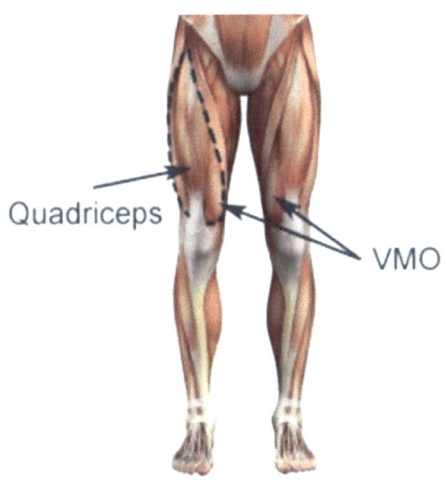

BEFORE TAPING THE PATELLA

➢ It is crucial to first find the harmed area where the bottom of the knee cap rubs on the tibia bone. The knee cap normally should be glided laterally away from the harmed area.

➢ The knee cap should be rotated or titled, moving it medially. The therapist should look and examine the patella. If your first effort is unsuccessful, then attempt another tilt or rotation.

➢ The usefulness of taping needs to be examined by executing an activity which normally triggers pain just before applying the tape, which can be then repeated once the tape is applied. In case the taping is helpful then the activity must be almost pain free.

➢ Clean your skin before applying the tape. What this means is no oils, or lotions of any type. You want the skin to be thoroughly clean and most importantly dry. Moisture of any type will cause the tape to fall off.

➢ Preferably, the less hair the better. This means that for ideal results you'll have to cut any long hair on the leg or shave the calf area.

➢ The tape must last 4-5 days. You can shower with it on. Only towel dry it after shower. You don't need to use a hair dryer, the tape is heat activated.

HOW TO TAPE

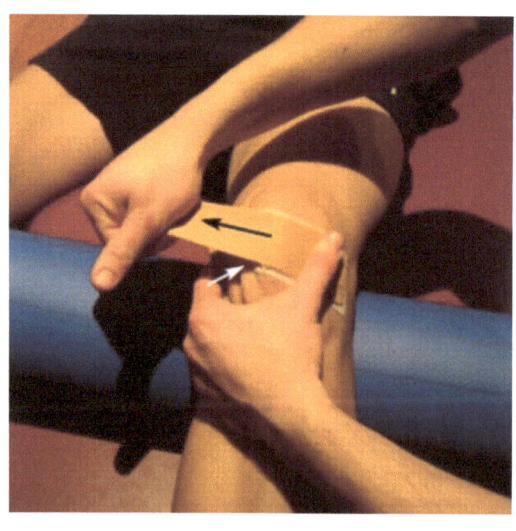

➢Get started lying down on your back, with the knee a little bit curved, but fully relaxed and a foam roller or towel underneath the knee.

➢Start the tape in line with the center of the knee cap at the outside part of the knee.

➢ Making use of your thumb on the top of the sports tape, carefully press the knee cap to the inside part of the knee while making use of your fingers to drag the skin at the inner part of the knee to the knee cap.

➢ Finish off this taping method at the inner part of the knee making sure you've made some wrinkles in the skin at the inner part of the knee. Repeat the method 2-3 times, according to the amount of support needed.

REMOVING THE TAPE

Care must be taken when removing the tape to prevent skin damage. The tape needs to be taken off slowly and gradually, tugging the tape back on itself with pressure inserted on the skin close to the line of attachment of the tape. Usually tape must be taken off within 48 hours or earlier if there's any raise in pain or symptoms.

CONCLUSION

Thank you for reading this book!

I hope this book was able to help you to deal with your patellofemoral pain syndrome effectively.

The next step is to remember your fitness routines and continue them.

Thank you and good luck!

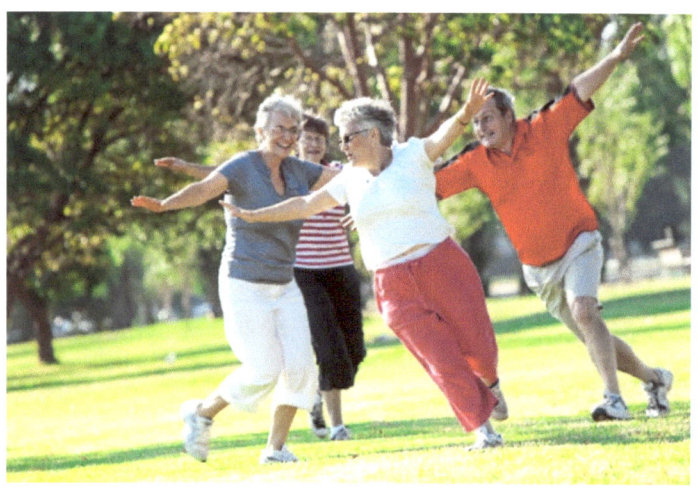

www.ingramcontent.com/pod-product-compliance
Lightning Source LLC
Chambersburg PA
CBHW050838290526
45792CB00001B/441